A User's Guide to
A BETTER BOD

*Wisdom for Facing the Trials of
a Healthier, Happier You*

Jo Elder and M.I. Wiser

Ilustrations by Janora Bayot

One More Press
Lake Oswego, Oregon

Printed in the United States of America.

Copyright © 1992 by Jo Elder & M.I. Wiser

Library of Congress Cataloging-in-Publication Data

Elder, Jo -
    A user's guide to a better bod: wisdom for facing the trials of
creating a healthier, happier you/by Jo Elder and M.I. Wiser.
        p .   cm.
    ISBN 0-941361-96-9 : $6.50
    1.Health. 2. Reducing. 3. Body image   I. Wiser, M.I.,
    II. Title.
RA776.5.E43   1992
613.2'5—dc20   92-21172
                                                               CIP

One More Press
P.O. Box 1885
Lake Oswego, OR 97035
(503) 697-7964

A User's Guide to A Better Bod

Introduction

You only get one body, and it's supposed to last a lifetime. But nobody bothers to give you an operator's manual, so when the darn thing starts to fall apart, you don't have the slightest idea what went wrong. Think of **A User's Guide to A Better Bod** as your operator's manual!

Oh, you think you don't need a set of instructions? You say you've been getting by all these years without one? Well, spend a few minutes buck-naked in front of a full length mirror and you'll see little resemblance to those streamlined images that entice you into buying everything from soft drinks to new jeans. Yet deep down you know you think buying their products will make you more like them.

Compare that body of yours to the new car you've been drooling over. It'll have an operator's manual in the glove box, and one of the first things you'll do is read it. After all, that's where you'll find out how to keep it running smoothly, which kind of gasoline to use, when to change the oil and how to diagnose problems.

A User's Guide to A Better Bod does the same thing for your body. It'll teach you how to laugh at the problems involved in struggling with the perfect body image, what it takes to keep your body running smoothly, which are the best foods for optimum performance, how exercise is like changing the oil, and why many of today's health problems are related to poor body maintenance.

In short, as you read this guide, you'll learn exactly what changes you need to make in order to keep your body operating as well as it should for as long as possible.

Stop letting your body make all the decisions, take charge of your life, and begin treating your body like the highly-tuned piece of equipment it is. You'll be glad you did!

Jo Elder
M. I. Wiser

Important Note: Always check with your doctor before beginning any new exercise or weight-loss program, especially if you have health problems or are severely overweight.

To all of you who wage the war
to better your body against what seems to be
a never-ending series of temptations.

1 ☺ You can't control your weight if
      you don't take charge of your life.

2 ☺ *"He who does not mind his belly will
      hardly mind anything else."*
                              Samuel Johnson

3 ☺ Change your body image for
      yourself, not someone else.

4 ☺ Building your confidence and self-esteem is the first step in improving your body image.

5 ☺ Stop worrying about what other people think about your body.

6 ☺ Love yourself no matter what size you happen to be.

7 ☺ *"No man can make you feel inferior without your consent."*
                                Eleanor Roosevelt

8 ☺ Believe in yourself! Start each day by looking your mirror image in the eye and saying, "I have control over my life and can do anything I set out to do."

9 ☺ The most important part of a successful weight-loss program is a good mental attitude.

10 ☺ Develop a sense of humor. So what if some fool laughs at you because you're overweight. You can always lose weight but they're stuck with a lousy attitude.

11 ☺ Losing weight is not an act of vanity, it's a move toward creating a healthier body.

12 ☺ Maintaining your proper body weight will reduce the wear and tear on your joints.

13 ☺ Listen to your body.

14 ☺ Don't just go on a diet. The key to a successful weight-loss program is to change your eating habits.

15 ☺ To lose weight, you simply have to burn more calories than you eat.

16 ☺ Regular exercise is a great appetite suppressant.

17 ☺ People who exercise regularly require less sleep.

18 ☺ Regular exercise will trim your body faster than eating less food.

19 ☺ Running, biking, skiing, swimming and other aerobic exercises are big calorie burners.

20 ☺ You can increase your metabolism with regular exercise and good healthy eating habits.

21 ☺ Develop an "elevator phobia" – always take the stairs, even if only part of the way.

22 ☺ Walking will keep you young.

23 ☺ Yard work is a great calorie burner. Weeding the garden burns 440 calories per hour, mowing the lawn 396, trimming hedges 270 and raking leaves 192.

24 ☺ Counting calories is not enough, the kind of food you eat is just as important as how many calories.

25 ☺ Believe in yourself! If you set your mind to creating a slimmer body, you know you can make it happen.

26 ☺ Most overweight people are on a *seefood* diet, they see food so they eat. Put yourself on a *leavefood* diet, make a point of leaving food on your plate.

27 ☺ Exercise is the key to good health.

28 ☺ A good way to reduce your appetite is by drinking generous amounts of water.

29 ☺ *"Water, taken in moderation, cannot hurt anybody."*

Mark Twain

30 ☺ Pets give unconditional approval, they don't care how you look, and make wonderful exercise partners.

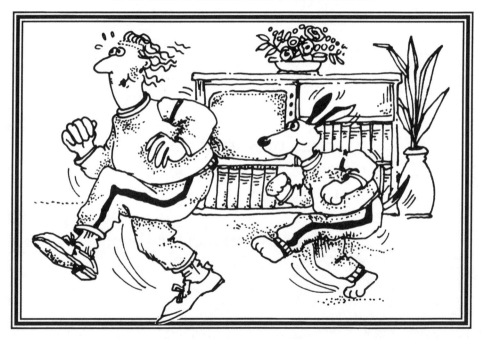

31 ☺ *"A full belly makes a dull brain."*
　　　　　　　　　　　Benjamin Franklin

32 ☺ Exercise preserves muscle. With exercise, weight loss means fat lost.

33 ☺ Fat is fat and muscle is muscle and never the twain shall meet.

34 ☺ Join an exercise group.

35 ☺ Cycling is a good overall body conditioner. The act of pedaling builds strength in your buttocks, calves and thighs.

36 ☺ Avoid people who tempt you from your goals.

37 ☺ Always drink lots of liquids before and during exercise.

38 ☺ A daily walking program will tone flabby muscles, give you energy and help you to lose weight without dieting.

39 ☺ Can't jog? Try skipping.

40 ☺ One low-exercise way to reduce fat is to stop opening the refrigerator.

41 ☺ *"Doesn't thou love life? Then do not squander time, for that is the stuff life is made of."*

Benjamin Franklin

42 ☺ Fat cells choke your heart.

43 ☺ Fat people are likely candidates for high blood pressure, diabetes, heart disease, kidney trouble, circulatory disorders, hernias, arthritis and gallstones.

44 ☺ Instead of counting calories, focus on eating lowfat, high-fiber, high-carbohydrate foods.

45 ☺ *"When you have to make a choice and don't make it, that in itself is a choice."*

William James

46 ☺ A diet that doesn't require dieting, or an exercise plan that requires no exercise, is only for the reducer who doesn't really want to reduce.

47 ☺ Make time for the important things in life. Exercise is one of them.

48 ☺ Choose an exercise activity you enjoy and you'll have a much better chance of sticking to it.

49 ☺ Find a hobby, like swimming or tennis, that requires exercise.

50 ☺ Pushing yourself to the point of pain when exercising only injures the muscles you're trying to help.

51 ☺ It's just as important to give your body quality rest as it is to give it a quality workout.

52 ☺ Join a volkswalking group.

53 ☺ If you hate exercise, start simple.
Do a few each morning until it
becomes a habit, then increase the
number of repetitions.

54 ☺ If you've never exercised, don't
start out with a five-day-a-week
program, begin with a 20-minute
walk.

55 ☺ Avoid anything that's been fried, creamed, sauteed or battered.

56 ☺ *"At a dinner party one should eat wisely but not too well, and talk well but not too wisely."*
W. Somerset Maugham

57 ☺ Take charge of your eating habits.

58 ☺ Never stand near the buffet table.

59 ☺ Fat people tend to wolf down their food; thin people seem to take their time. Eat slowly!

60 ☺ Enjoy your food. Focus on the color, taste, aroma and texture. Linger over each bite.

61 ☺ Don't be surprised if you feel hungry all the time when you begin your diet change. You're fighting a lifetime of habits.

62 ☺ Never eat in front of the TV.

63 ☺ Learn to control the things that lead you to overeat.

64 ☺ Humankind was given a sense of humor to make up for nature's law of gravity.

65 ☺ It's never too late to get your body back into condition.

66 ☺ See your doctor before beginning any new weight-loss program.

67 ☺ Don't say "I should work out" or "I should skip dessert"; say "I will exercise because I want to feel better" or "I'll skip dessert because I want to be slim". *Should* makes you feel deprived; *want* will make you feel good about yourself.

68 ☺ Take up rollerskating.

69 ☺ Slow walking is better than no walking, but fast walking is even better.

70 ☺ Do this exercise at your desk or in the car. Sit up straight and suck in your tummy muscles in as hard as you can. Breathe out and hold for five seconds. Repeat until tired.

71 ☺ While washing dishes or running the vacuum, suck in your tummy muscles and clench your buttocks together. Hold this for 10 seconds, breathing normally. Repeat as often as you can.

72 ☺ Walking four times a week will help prevent osteoporosis.

73 ☺ Place encouraging notes around the house for an extra boost. Put them on the refrigerator door, next to the cookie jar, in the freezer and beside the bathroom scale.

🐾 A User's Guide to A Better Bod 🐾

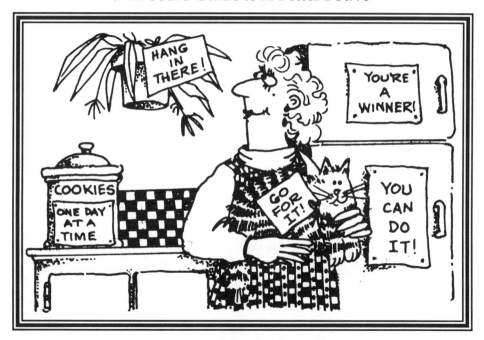

74 ☺ Walkers who carry hand weights burn more calories.

75 ☺ The reason most people don't stick to a new weight-loss program is because they go into it with unrealistic expectations. If you think your program is easy and fun, you'll probably stick with it.

76 ☺ Losing weight won't solve all your problems.

77 ☺ People who think positive thoughts about themselves are more successful at losing weight.

78 ☺ Exercise causes the body's HDL (good cholesterol) to rise.

79 ☺ Nothing is either good or bad but by comparison.

80 ☺ Control your appetite by putting your fork down between bites. When eating sandwiches, set the sandwich down between bites.

81 ☺ Drink lowfat or skim milk.

82 ☺ Drink a glass of skim or lowfat milk half an hour before a meal. It will make you feel full.

83 ☺ Use low-calorie salad dressing.

84 ☺ In restaurants, ask for your salad dressing on the side so you can control the amount you use.

85 ☺ Try cutting out just one dessert a week rather than swearing off desserts for life. You'll have a better chance for success and can easily double your commitment in the second week.

86 ☺ Most dieters will benefit from a good daily multiple vitamin.

87 ☺ Dieting is a trying time when you stop eating food and start eating calories.

88 ☺ *"An empty stomach is not a good political adviser."*

Albert Einstein

89 ☺ Be a good loser!

90 ☺ A proper diet includes 25 grams or more of fiber each day.

91 ☺ If you increase your fiber consumption too fast you may experience cramps, gas or bloating.

92 ☺ Long-grain brown rice has three times as much fiber as white rice.

93 ☺ Limit meat to no more than 4 ounces a day.

94 ☺ Choose your chicken or turkey wisely; the thigh has the most fat and the breast the least.

95 ☺ Cut down on fat. This includes red meats, fried foods and cheese.

96 ☺ Dieting is always difficult, but making healthy changes in your lifestyle can be fun.

97 ☺ Counting calories is tedious. It's easier to practice healthy eating.

98 ☺ Diets that rely on just one food, such as grapefruit, are not healthy.

99 ☺ Do you eat when you're unhappy?
Are you unhappy because you're
fat? It's a never-ending cycle.

100 ☺ Drink 8 glasses of water every day.

101 ☺ No person is really fat; he is either
too heavy for his height, or too
short for his weight.

102 ☺ Learn to reward yourself in a non-food way. Indulge yourself by going shopping, for a massage, a facial or some other "feel good" activity.

103 ☺ Instead of raiding the refrigerator during commercials, why not burn calories with 3 minutes of exercise.

104 ☺ Be realistic. No matter what you do, life will still have its ups and downs. Don't let the downs lead you into self-pity or binges.

105 ☺ Exercise reduces fat. Exercising your stomach (eating) does not.

106 ☺ Never eat someone else's leftovers.

107 ☺ If you lose weight too fast, you'll wind up walking around inside skin that doesn't fit.

108 ☺ It's not losing weight that's the problem. It's losing it in a way that it won't come back.

109 ☺ Miracles don't happen overnight.

110 ☺ Make it a habit never to eat between meals.

111 ☺ Never eat out of a container. Serve yourself a small portion and put the container back before eating.

112 ☺ There's no such thing as a harmless junk food snack.

113 ☺ Think of your body as a highly tuned race car. It can't run on empty and performs its best on high quality fuel.

114 ☺ The place to improve your eating habits is in the supermarket. Good planning can make an enormous difference in the way you eat.

115 ☺ A lot of men claim they wear the same size pants they wore in high school when in fact they're just wearing them lower and letting it all hang over the top.

116 ☺ When you go to a smaller size, get rid of your "big" clothes. Saving them only reinforces self-doubt.

117 ☺ More diets start in dress shops
than in doctors' offices.

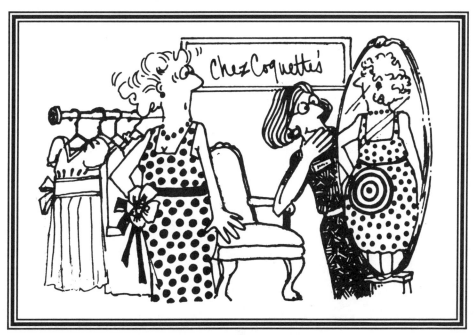

118 ☺ Don't eat everything on your plate.

119 ☺ Pasta isn't fattening, but the meatballs, sauce and cheese are. Find a low-calorie topping.

120 ☺ Never eat in bed.

121 ☺ Chew each bite 40 times.

122 ☺ Don't eat after dinner.

123 ☺ Always eat at the dinner table.

124 ☺ Make diet meals festive by using your good china and candlelight.

125 ☺ Overweight people eat more dietary fat than lean people.

126 ☺ Being overweight is sometimes caused by glands, but more often by those muscles that enable you to reach for second helpings.

127 ☺ Retrain your taste buds. Buy lean cuts of meat, substitute frozen yogurt for ice cream, and use low-fat salad dressing.

128 ☺ Always take a break between drinks, whether it's alcohol or anything else besides water.

129 ☺ Making a commitment to improve your body is very empowering.

130 ☺ Overeating is destructive. Learn to stop when you're full.

131 ☺ If you keep losing and regaining weight it gets harder each time because without exercise you're losing muscle mass but gaining fat. Exercise makes weight loss fat loss.

132 ☺ Ballroom dancing is fun and burns 180 calories per hour while toning muscles.

133 ☺ Even 10-minute exercise stints will pay off if done regularly.

134 ☺ If you have to gasp for breath while doing aerobic exercises, you're going too fast.

135 ☺ Make exercising an event rather than a chore.

136 ☺ The more muscle mass you have, the more calories you will burn doing absolutely nothing.

137 ☺ Spend at least five minutes on warm-up exercises before beginning any vigorous exercise.

138 ☺ Try jumping rope.

139 ☺ Lie on your back with your feet flat on the floor and your hands folded behind your head. Lift your head and shoulders off the floor and hold for five seconds while squeezing your tummy muscles tightly. Slowly lower your head and shoulders. Repeat at least five times.

140 ☺ Lie on your back with your knees bent, feet on the floor. Bring your right knee up to your chest, hold for two seconds and lower. Repeat with left knee. Do 10 to 15 sets.

141 ☺ Take a health spa vacation.

142 ☺ Never use the drive-up window.

143 ☺ Walking won't build your endurance for other activities, but it will help you to lose weight while helping your heart.

144 ☺ Walking, running, cycling and other weight-bearing exercises can slow the natural effects of aging on muscles and joints.

145 ☺ When sitting in a chair, lift your right foot off the floor a few inches and hold for 10 seconds. Repeat with the other foot. Do these anytime you're watching TV, or while at your desk.

146 ☺ Alcohol consumption adds empty calories.

147 ☺ Eat a salad before going to a party where you'll find tempting foods.

148 ☺ If you brush your teeth often, you'll fool your mouth into thinking you've already eaten.

149 ☺ Being overweight affects your general health.

150 ☺ Don't be one of those people who tells others how slim they once were; concentrate on how slim you're going to be.

151 ☺ Never resign yourself to being fat. You'll start out a *before*, become a *during*, and with lots of effort, you'll someday be an *after*.

152 ☺ Frustration is the difference between what you are and what you think you are.

153 ☺ Admit your failures then get back on your diet.

154 ☺ Don't use your weight as an excuse for life's problems.

155 ☺ Heredity has its limits; quit blaming your heritage for your weight problem.

156 ☺ Imagine you're 20 pounds lighter. Work off those 20 pounds before setting your next body image.

157 ☺ Keep a journal.

158 ☺ Lean body mass declines with increasing age. 60-year-olds who weigh the same as they did at age 20 need fewer calories, but the need for nutrients is not less.

159 ☺ Measure your success by how your body feels and how your clothes fit, not by your body weight.

160 ☺ Never wear clothing that's too small. It'll make you look larger and could give way, creating an embarassing situation.

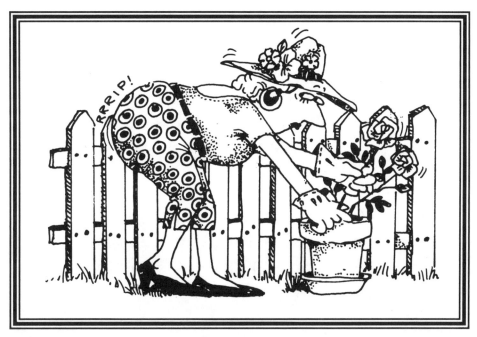

161 ☻ Make good eating habits a family goal. A person who sits on the couch munching chips cannot expect others in the household to go without.

162 ☻ Overeaters have lots in common; extra chins, love handles, spare tires, low energy and early death.

163 ☺ Paddle your own canoe, both physically and spiritually. The first will give you exercise, the second will allow you to choose your own image rather than one that's sold by advertisers.

164 ☺ If a diet sounds too good to be true, it is.

165 ☻ What many people call aging is little more than the accumulation of a lifetime of inactivity which has caused muscles to shrink and body fat to increase.

166 ☻ Whether it's 5 pounds, 30 pounds, or 150 pounds, the majority of people are overweight.

167 ☺ Exercise increases your metabolic rate and reduces your appetite.

168 ☺ Once you increase your metabolic rate, weight loss is easier.

169 ☺ The average person's metabolic rate drops by 10 to 15% while watching 30 minutes of TV.

170 ☺ Extremely hot or cold weather will increase your metabolic rate by up to 10%. Lower the thermostat in the winter and shut off the air conditioner in the summer for an extra fat-burning boost.

171 ☺ People who fidgit burn up to 500 extra calories a day

172 ☺ Aerobic exercise can keep your metabolic rate boosted for about 24 hours.

173 ☺ Keep fresh fruit on the table.

174 ☺ Apples are great for curbing your appetite. Find a variety you like and keep some handy.

175 ☺ Air-popped popcorn has 1/3 fewer calories than normal popcorn, and supplies 1.5 grams of fiber per cup.

176 ☺ Don't fall into the pattern of thinking of yourself as either being "on" or "off" your diet.

177 ☺ Banish junk food from your home.

178 ☺ Drink water. Many people get over half their calories through liquid intake. Fruit drinks, juices, sodas, milk, sweetened coffee or tea and alcoholic drinks all add calories.

179 ☺ Eat 25% of your daily caloric intake for breakfast, 50% for lunch and 25% for dinner.

180 ☺ If you can't stomach the thought of food early in the day, try a mid-morning snack. It'll keep the hunger monster under control.

181 ☺ You don't have to win every battle.

182 ☺ Fresh fruit has little or no fat, cholesterol or sodium.

183 ☺ Fresh berries are very low in calories yet will satisfy sugar cravings and supply fiber. Papaya, cantaloupe, strawberries, oranges, tangerines, kiwis, mangos, persimmons, watermelon, raspberries, grapefruit and blackberries are among the most nutritious.

184 ☺ *"One should eat to live, not live to eat."*

Moliere

185 ☺ A gram of fat contains 9 calories; a gram of carbohydrate or protein contains only 4 calories. You can eat more carbohydrates than fats without adding extra calories.

186 ☺ If you can lay off the salt and sweets for just 30 days, your taste buds will begin to enjoy the subtle variety in healthy foods and you'll lose the craving.

187 ☺ *"I can resist everything except temptation."*

Oscar Wilde

188 ☺ After filling your plate, wrap up all the leftovers and put them in the freezer. This is a great way to keep yourself from having seconds.

189 ☺ Eat wisely.

190 ☺ Replace red meat with chicken, fish or turkey as often as you can.

191 ☺ Limit fat consumption to less than 25 percent of your daily calories.

192 ☺ Buy yourself a nice selection of lowfat cookbooks.

193 ☺ Choose broth soups over cream soups, and limit your crackers to just a few.

194 ☺ Celebrate each 5-pound loss in a non-food way.

195 ☺ Start your morning by imagining yourself shopping for clothes one size smaller than you currently wear.

196 ☺ Eat 25 to 35 grams of fiber daily.

197 ☺ Buy in small quantitites. 'Penny wise' is 'pound foolish' when you buy jumbo-size junk food.

198 ☺ Fiber is a great weight-loss tool. Put lots of vegetables, fruits and whole grains in your diet.

199 ☺ Gimmicky diets don't work.

200 ☺ Make "off limits" foods hard to get
at. Keep them frozen or in a
difficult-to-reach place.

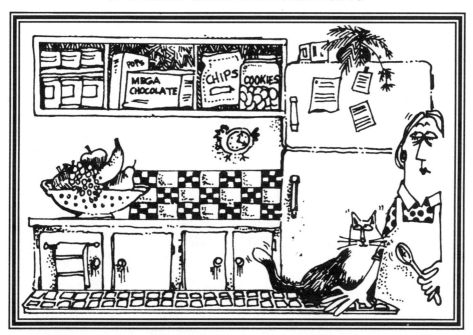

201 ☺ Eat just 14 potato chips and you'll use up 15% of your daily fat limit. And just how many of us stop at 14 chips?

202 ☺ *"In general, mankind, since the improvement of cookery, eat twice as much as nature requires."*
Benjamin Franklin

203 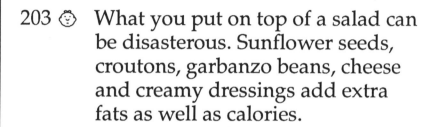 What you put on top of a salad can be disasterous. Sunflower seeds, croutons, garbanzo beans, cheese and creamy dressings add extra fats as well as calories.

204 Undercooked vegetables are healthier – fewer nutrients escape in the cooking process.

205 ☺ Water fills you up and brings a healthy glow to your skin.

206 ☺ If you eat the bulk of your calories early in the day, you'll have more time to burn them off. Whatever you eat right before bedtime will almost certainly turn to fat because your activity level is low.

207 ☺ Populations that eat fiber-rich foods have lower rates of colon cancer.

208 ☺ Read labels carefully! The recommended daily intake for cholesterol is only 300 mg yet many canned foods contain more than that in just one small can.

209 ☺ Creamed vegetables are fattening.

210 ☺ As you lose weight it helps to update your appearance. After losing 20 pounds, you'll want to get some more fashionable clothes, a new hairstyle or go for a cosmetic makeover. It's a new body and it deserves a new look.

211 ☺ If you loosen your belt during a meal, you're eating too much.

212 ☺ Never start a weight-loss program during a high-stress time of life.

213 ☺ It's easier to acquire two good habits than to break off one bad one.

214 ☺ *"The chains of habit are too weak to be felt until they are too strong to be broken."*

Samuel Johnson

215 ☺ If you have a choice between exerting energy and taking the easy route, always exert the energy.

216 ☺ Most people can dramatically lower their blood pressure by losing ten pounds and using less salt.

217 ☺ Beware of sodium additives when purchasing prepared foods. If sodium is part of any word, it will contribute to your sodium intake.

218 ☺ Use a salt substitute. Take the salt shaker off both the table and stove.

219 ☺ Keep air-popped, unbuttered popcorn in your cookie jar.

220 ☺ Be sure you're eating a balanced diet. You need to eat from all four food groups every day.

221 ☺ Don't munch while cooking.

222 ☺ Mealtimes should never be piggybacked onto other activities. Give them their separate time and place.

223 ☺ Make meat a side dish rather than a main dish.

224 ☺ *"Blame is a lazy man's wages"*
Danish proverb

225 ☺ You're not a failure if you fall off
your diet, you're simply human.
Tomorrow is another day.

226 ☺ You have to love yourself before
you can expect others to love you.

227 ☺ A sensible weight loss is 2 pounds per week. Anything more dramatic and you'll probably put the weight back on just as soon as you slip off your diet.

228 ☺ Salad dressing, margarine, cheese and ground beef are the number one source of fats in most diets.

229 ☺ Seafood is lower in saturated fat than skinless chicken breast.

230 ☺ Salmon and halibut are higher in calories than cod, haddock, abalone or tuna.

231 ☺ Raw carrots have only 45 calories per cup.

232 ☺ A pound of radishes has just 50 calories.

233 ☺ Raw vegetables require more chewing and stimulate your brain, making you feel fuller.

234 ☺ Use low-fat cottage cheese instead of ricotta when making lasagne.

235 ☺ The first thing most people lose on a new diet is their sense of humor.

236 ☺ Be wary of setting unrealistic goals. It only leads to failure and guilt.

237 ☺ Broil, bake, roast or boil your food. Don't fry!

238 ☺ Before you go out to dinner, eat a piece of fruit or other lowfat snack. If you're starving by the time you see food, you'll overdo.

239 ☺ In restaurants, always have gravies and sauces served on the side. Make it your goal to use less than half of whatever they bring you.

240 ☺ Organize a diet support group.

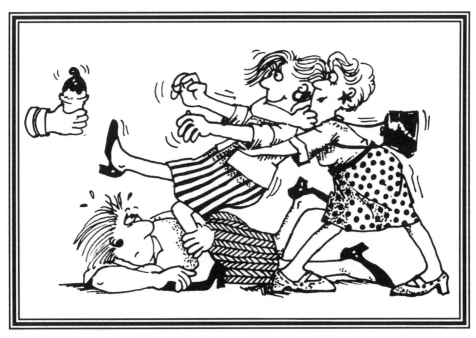

241 ☺ Read food labels carefully. Ingredients are listed according to weight, so major ingredients are listed first. Watch out for items like sugar: they are often listed under several different names.

242 ☺ Trim all fat from meat before cooking.

243 ☺ The best way to lower your cholesterol is to eat less saturated fat.

244 ☺ When farmers want to fatten up their pigs they feed them fats. You're doing the same thing to your body when you eat a diet that's high in fats. Oink, oink!

245 ☺ Invest in a good non-stick pan and you'll use less fat.

246 ☺ Substitute yogurt in dishes calling for sour cream or mayonnaise.

247 ☺ A fresh flower at your place setting makes a low-calorie meal high in appeal.

248 ☺ Since digestion burns calories, and so does exercise, it makes good sense that a 20-minute walk after dinner will work wonders.

249 ☺ You won't be ticketed for exceeding the "feed limit", but that doesn't mean you won't pay a penalty.

250 ☺ The next time you're craving food, try drinking a cup of water instead. Sometimes your body will send you "hunger" messages when it's really only thirsty.

251 ☺ Whenever possible, substitute a low-calorie drink for a high-calorie one.

252 ☺ It takes 20 minutes for your brain to get the message that it's full. The slower you eat, the less chance you have of overeating.

253 ☺ Instead of sauteing in butter, use a bit of broth or vegetable oil. Most good restaurants will substitute this method when requested.

254 ☺ One good way to reduce is by exercising your will power.

255 ☺ Fill your candy dish with marbles.

256 ☺ Adults are people who have stopped growing vertically and are now expanding their horizontal space.

257 ☺ Reduce your sugar. Sugar stimulates your appetite by disrupting your insulin/blood sugar balance and results in cravings for the wrong kinds of foods.

258 ☺ Have a mental image of yourself as an energetic, healthy, trim person.

259 ☺ Stress makes you eat quickly.

260 ☺ Soft music played at meal time will help you to eat slowly. You'll find yourself savoring each bite as you savor the calming sound of music.

261 ☺ There is no such thing as a harmless junk food snack.

262 ☺ Say "yes" to positive actions. If you
always blow your diet when
eating out, make a game out of
putting "restaurant dollars" away
for a new wardrobe or vacation.

263 ☺ There's nothing jolly about
overweight people who can't bend
over to tie their own shoes.

264 ☺ Think of your body as occupying a definite space. Visualize a slim space for yourself.

265 ☺ The fat on your body is simply the result of eating more calories than you burn off.

266 ☺ Most casseroles are high in fat.

267 ☺ *"The only way to keep your health is to eat what you don't want, drink what you don't like and do what you'd rather not."*

Mark Twain

268 ☺ Buy extra-lean ground beef and save 400 to 700 calories per pound over regular ground beef.

269 ☺ Cooked fresh yams are filling, loaded with fiber and have only 80 calories. Leave off the butter.

270 ☺ Avoid ready-to-serve foods, they're loaded with extra calories.

271 ☺ Holiday foods can be a dietary killer. Practice self control.

272 ☺ Use a smaller plate.

273 ☺ A higher metabolic rate produces more body heat and reduces your appetite.

274 ☺ It's not the half hour you spend at the table that adds weight, it's the seconds.

275 ☺ People who skip breakfast or lunch generally binge after dinner.

276 ☺ Skipping meals drains your energy level and makes it harder to resist tempting foods later.

277 ☺ The more varieties of food served at a meal, the more you'll eat.

278 ☺ Use cornstarch to thicken sauces, instead of flour, and save calories. Although cornstarch contains more calories per tablespoon, you use less of it.

279 ☺ You can save yourself 120 calories just by removing the skin from your chicken breast.

280 ☺ Walk to the grocery store – you can't carry much back.

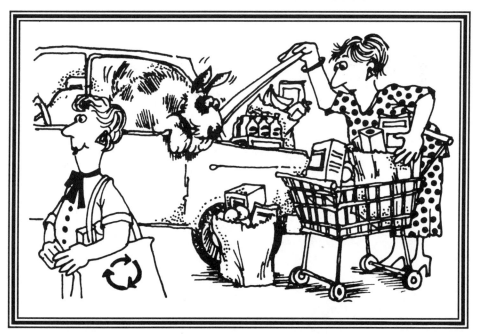

281 ☺ There are approximately 13 teaspoons of sugar products in a 12-ounce can of pop.

282 ☺ When trying to lose weight, high-fat foods should be the first thing you eliminate. They probably contribute the most to your weight problem.

283 ☺ When eating out, look for heart-healthy items. Once you learn the rules of healthy eating you'll find them easy to spot.

284 ☺ A good rule to remember, when it comes to eating, is that you can generally help yourself more by helping yourself to less.

285 ☺ The earlier in the day you eat high-calorie items, the more time you have to burn them off.

286 ☺ When you reduce your caloric intake, your metabolism slows down. Exercise is essential or else you're starving yourself for nothing.

287 ☺ To learn how many pounds your favorite "bad" food adds each year write down the number of calories it contains, multiply this by the number of times you eat it in an average week, multiply by 52 and divide by 3,500. The resulting number is how many pounds you'll gain if you keep it up.

288 ☺ Be realistic about your favorite foods. You're bound to fail if you say you'll **never** eat them again. Instead, tell yourself you'll only eat those foods on special occasions, and in moderation.

289 ☺ You really have to want to change before you'll find success.

290 ☺ Purchase a good home video exercise tape. Your authors' favorites are Richard Simmons' *Sweatin' to the Oldies®* and anything by Jane Fonda.

291 ☺ Stand in front of a full-length mirror, stark naked, to get yourself motivated.

292 😊 Before you sit down to a holiday feast, spend five minutes in front of the bathroom mirror, eye-to-eye with your image outlining exactly what you will and will not put on your plate. A small helping of dessert makes the perfect reward.

293 😊 Never give up!

294 ☺ Being honest about how long it took you to put on your extra weight will help you to be realistic about how fast it will come off.

295 ☺ Don't put your weight-loss plans off until after the holidays, your birthday, someone's party, etc. Start today!

296 ☺ If you use more than one napkin during a meal, you're eating too much of the wrong kind of food.

297 ☺ Know what triggers your over-eating: vacations, cooking for guests, high-stress deadlines, etc. If you're aware of the causes, it's easier to fortify your willpower.

298 ☺ Foods high in carbohydrates turn off your hunger while high-fat foods turn on your cravings for more fats.

299 ☺ As you exercise, teach your mind to isolate the muscles you want to work. Visualize these muscles before, during and after exercise.

300 ☺ Don't kid yourself into thinking that you already get enough exercise. If you're overweight, you're not getting enough exercise.

301 ☺ Watching TV burns 72 calories an hour, ironing 114, cleaning the house 210 and fast dancing 366. Learn to combine activities.

302 ☺ Give yourself permission to indulge once in a while. Denial often leads to binges.

303 ☺ Park as far away from any appointment as you can and walk.

304 ☺ When making gravy, skim off the fat first for a healthier gravy.

305 ☺ A small tomato has only 25 calories and provides lots of fiber.

306 ☺ One half of what we eat enables us to live; the other half enables the doctor to live.

307 ☺ Do not resent growing old; many are denied the privilege.

308 ☺ *"I wish to preach, not the doctrine of
ignoble ease, but the doctrine of the
strenuous life."*
                          Theodore Roosevelt

309 ☺ Don't let bad weather ruin your
walking habit. Take it inside. Try
the mall, airport terminal or some
other large building.

310 ☺ Become a volunteer at your local hospital. If you can help out by delivering flowers or magazines, you'll get in lots of walking.

311 ☺ Exercise releases endorphins into your bloodstream. This natural chemical will relieve pain, lift your spirits and decrease stress.

341 ☺ The more time you spend chewing,
the longer you'll feel full.

342 ☺ Even if you diet diligently, those
last few pounds are almost
impossible to remove. Keep in
mind: bodies that are this close to
perfection are judged perfect by
everyone but the owner.

312 ☺ *"Misleading are appearances. One's true self is within – a corpulent outside may hide a soul that's starved and thin."*

Rebecca McCann

313 ☺ One very effective diet consists of only four words: "No more, thank you!"

314 ☺ Do you eat every time you get bored? Find a hobby that is incompatible with eating.

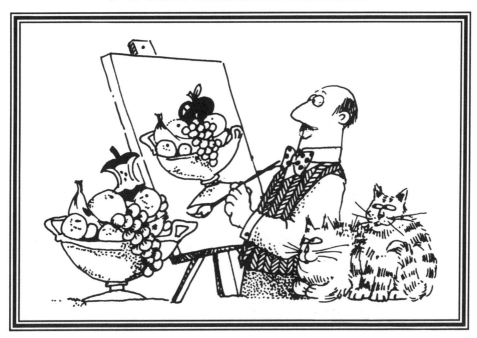

315 ☺ Never keep food anywhere but in the kitchen. That means no more snacks in the glove box, your desk, and especially in the bedroom!

316 ☺ Never take seconds of anything.

317 ☺ Don't shop for food when you're hungry. Always eat first.

318 Overeating is nothing more than a bad habit. Learn to keep your hands busy in the evening so you won't be using them to transport empty calories to your mouth.

319 People on diets lose weight not by talking about it, but by keeping their mouths shut.

320 ☺ Potatoes are an ideal weight loss food, they're loaded with fiber, potassium and low in calories. But lay off the sour cream and butter.

321 ☺ The best thing for a person on a diet to eat is – less.

322 ☺ Variety makes any diet easier.

323 ☺ Eating right might seem expensive, but nothing is more costly than poor health.

324 ☺ If breakfast is a meal you normally skip, try non-breakfast type foods.

325 ☺ If you make dinner your biggest meal, you'll never lose weight.

326 ☺ True adulthood is attained when you begin eating what is good for you, instead of eating whatever you like.

327 ☺ Genetics determine where your body will deposit fat, but you determine how much you'll allow your body to deposit.

328 ☺ Learn to poke fun at yourself.
When you catch yourself ordering
a hot fudge sundae, ask yourself if
it's really more satisfying than
having the trimmer body you've
been telling yourself you want.

329 ☺ It only takes 3,500 calories to add
one pound of fat.

330 😊 Make a list of all the benefits you'll get from losing weight and post it where you will see it often.

331 😊 Practice moderation. Too much of anything, except water, can cause your body harm.

332 😊 You can control your weight!

333 ☺ You don't have to eat everything brought to your table in restaurants. In fact, it's a good idea to send back the rolls, or at least send back the butter.

334 ☺ Make a list of all of the non-food items that bring you pleasure. Use them to replace munching.

335 ☺ Never eat while doing something else.

336 ☺ Quit eating before you're full. Overeating stretches your stomach muscles and you end up eating more each time. If you learn to stop eating before your stomach is full, you'll shrink your stomach.

ORDER COUPON

Please send:

___ A User's Guide to A Better Bod @ $6.50 ea.   _____
___ A User's Guide to Love @ $6.50 ea.   _____
___ A User's Guide to Parenthood @ $6.50 ea.   _____
___ A User's Guide to Old Age @ $6.50 ea.   _____
___ A User's Guide to Pets @ $6.50 ea.   _____
___ A User's Guide to Money @ $6.50 ea.   _____

                          Shipping   2.50
                          Total Enclosed   _____

Name _____

Address _____

City/State/Zip Code _____

Send this order coupon with your check to:
One More Press, P.O. Box 1885, Lake Oswego, Oregon 97035.

Half Wisdom *Half Wit*

Other titles in this series include:

A USER'S GUIDE TO LOVE
A USER'S GUIDE TO PARENTHOOD
A USER'S GUIDE TO OLD AGE
A USER'S GUIDE TO PETS
A USER'S GUIDE TO MONEY

To receive further information on these and other books by
Jo Elder and M. I. Wiser send your name and address to:
One More Press, P.O. Box 1885, Lake Oswego, Oregon 97035.

337 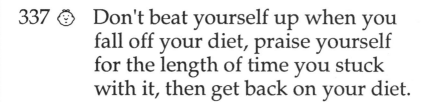 Don't beat yourself up when you fall off your diet, praise yourself for the length of time you stuck with it, then get back on your diet.

338 One of the best exercises you can do is to place your hands on the edge of the dinner table and push yourself back.

339 ☺ A healthy body is a lifetime commitment. Once you've reached your goal weight it's important to maintain a healthy diet and exercise program.

340 ☺ Snacking is your enemy; if you must snack eat raw vegetables or fresh fruit.